A Modern Pandemic
A blessing in disguise

By

Ravneet Kaur

And

Akira White

This is a story of a girl who went abroad nut higher education, but pandemic had different plans for her. She came back home in India during pandemic to stay at safe place however the isolation in times of pandemic changed her view of the world. She understood to achieve fulfilment in life it is important to work on inner engineering and the isolation period gave her opportunity to build a different perception on world and leave the career rat race behind

In this story book *"Pandemic 2020, A blessing in disguise"* Ravneet recounts her experiences in the new world where social distancing and staying at home was new normal. In her story she narrates about dealing with mental health and various techniques that helped her to stay calm and compose and later turned out to be a life changing factor for her

The Author

The author of this story is an ambitious Indian girl. Her story is based on the true experiences she faced during pandemic 2020. The stories are depiction of her realizing the value of privileges she has and how rich and poor are differentiated in her country. In addition, her story captures the ways the pandemic turned out to be a great learning experience for her in terms of emotional intelligence by consistent practice of medication and yoga.

She has been always enthusiastic about working towards community with lack of privileges. During pandemic she took the responsibility of making a change by helping every suffering person she can.

RAVNEET KAUR

The story of a girl surviving 2020 pandemic

It is 2020 and we all imagined the world full of flying cars and high buildings, AI territory but here we are locked inside our houses, no airplanes flying, no vehicle on roads, the world feels nothing less than a science fiction movie where our planet is taken over by aliens. But who imagined that a virus wouldn't be any less than alien? A small invisible creature who made the world turn upside down. It has been 6 months, and no one kissed under the Eifel tower, no one hiked in the Alaska, no streets are filled with musicians and dancers, no one go outside to eat anymore. But on the other hand, the earth started healing, the air became pure than ever before, the most polluted cities in the world saw stars for the first time, the nature was healing. I saw two rainbows in the sky, I have enjoyed all the three times of day, sunset hour became the most favourite hour of my day. Past few years people have been fighting for the climate crisis and stats were circulated regarding declaring the climate crisis a global emergency but no one imagined a virus would do what higher authorities could not. Its only been the third month since I am living in a lockdown, but the pollution rate has drastically reduced globally. Today each person on earth have outgrown their living rate at least by 10%. The world with 20 million cars on road and 1000 flights in air,

1 million people walking on streets, vendors selling vegetables and fruits, people chilling around in summers have come to the pause. No one would have ever imagined one day we would need more doctors and food providers in the world than any other successful entrepreneurs. The pandemic has proved that the lives we were living for past years, is not normal, normal is when our humanity, our earth is in harmony with our actions.

It all started in January of 2020, but on a very small scale. A lab in Wuhan accidently came across with deadly Virus, however the whole world was not informed about it and China tried to hide the affects of this virus for some time keeping WHO in loop. In January of 2020 there was no panic anywhere around the world and only very few people were aware about the virus during first few cases of infection. Therefore, I already planned to visit back my home in India, meet my best friends and my family. Meanwhile I also had plans to travel in North East part of country. At that point of time this was not declared as global health emergency. Its been a year since I am living in Berlin and I was very excited to visit home as planned for one month. I never thought I will be spending another five months at my home. This year I wanted to spend my summers in beautiful beaches of Spain, take scuba diving training but little did I know that this year travel will become nothing less than a dream. As planned, I packed my bags in month of February and left for India. I was meeting my boyfriend after 1 year, it is with him I had my trip planned to Sikkim, a north east part of India, for 6 days. I remember that was the last time I travelled since pandemic happened. We went to various places in Kolkata and Sikkim. There were tourists all around in the sightseeing places, lanes full of street food and almost all the places were very crowded. On our second last day in Sikkim, I heard people talking about the states banning tourists. I remember people were being evacuated from the hotels in Sikkim and no more tourists were allowed into the state. Those who were given two days of time to leave the state. There was chaos all around, it felt like a meteor was about to hit the Earth or world is ending. I remember my last time airport. Everyone face covered with masks, sanitizers being sprayed in the crowded places, people were distanced from each other, it felt like an episode of black mirror. Continuous news on internet explaining the infection created chaos in the world. Global pandemic was declared, international travels were banned. The very first wave of deadly virus was seen in Wuhan with thousands of people infected, making its way towards Europe. It broke me watching people killed by deadly virus back in my resident country. Germany being having the best health care system lost many people and another country in Europe, Spain saw the worst ever death rate since 1917. It took me a while to digest the news and on the other hand I was not myself sure if I am not the carrier coming from a European state.

The time I entered in India during February, there was no testing being done on the airports and as per the WHO the infection usually does not show up the symptoms for first 14 days. There was no way for me to get myself checked and the fact that I might infect other people too made me feel very helpless. The only repeated thought buzzing in my head was that I had travelled to two different states, met so many people on my way and if something happened to these people, I won't be able to forgive myself. After two days of fighting with my thoughts I came back home and decided to quarantine myself. During that time, we had a very famous festival called Holi, the festival of colors and all the house members, neighbors and friends visits each other's house to play with colors. At that time infection rate in India was very low, probably only 3 infected people were reported in the data, therefore no one considered it to be a big deal. No matter how much I avoided to go out and be in contact with people, my acquaintances forced to play Holi. By this time, I already encountered 30 people from my neighborhood. There were no symptoms showing up in my body until then therefore I tried to stay calm and contained. After few days, I was finally convinced that the infection has not reached me since no symptoms showed up. At that time WHO was giving regular updates on identifying the virus and out of that one update was regarding the inability to identify symptoms. This update again put me in the state of helplessness and finally I decided to inform health authorities and arrange testing for me. I was tested negative and this was the first time I saw panic and anxiety leaving my body. The survivors who were tested positive for virus were sharing their stories via internet. The disease made people exhausted physically to mentally.

The first few days are just mild fever and coughing followed by breathing problems after few days. The entire period of the infection exhausts person emotionally being isolated from their family members and friends. There were some people who were at a strict need of ventilators and few people just got better by some medicines and self-isolating them for a specific period. The health care workers were dealing with this sickness for the first and they were trying their best to save thousands of people at same time. The tendency of disease to kill some people mainly people in the category of 60+ threatened the nations with high population of senior citizen. Spain was one of them, in every first month 500000 people were dead and there was not a place left to bury them and their family members were hold off to perform any funeral rituals as well.

On the other hand I felt very lucky being at home with my family and also at that time there were just two and three cases in India but no was safe, we all knew it will make its way to India as well very soon and few days later it happened. There were few thousand cases in India, people coming from abroad were not been screened initially and this lead to spread of Virus. Very soon India declared lockdown and made quarantine compulsory for people coming from abroad. The government established no movement rule across the nation. Police force were allocated at almost every street. Its been months now since the countries have been declared the lockdown and its not coming to end very soon. Just a day before lockdown I visited my school friends after 6 years and we have not been able to see other since months now. We celebrated birthday of a friend and slept over little did we knew that we won't be meeting again even after the fact that houses were only few miles apart.

First week of hearing the news of lockdown was very hard on me personally. Being a person who is always on a go, the idea of being captured at one place makes me feel agitated. I started fighting with my sibling, my parents, I felt very lost at that time. I remember waking up a day and watching news about virus filled me with so much of negativity, I cried for whole day. I knew this is going to be very difficult for me, I knew anxiety, depression, mental health issues were making their ways into our lives. More than the virus, loneliness was about to hit many youngsters. Our generation Is restless, we work hard and party harder. Our weekends are occupied with social gatherings, evenings over drink with strangers, we hardly stay at a place for so long. I knew life is going to be this way for some time and I must prepare myself to deal with it. Just when I started accepting the situation, I felt a very strange behavior from my boyfriend side. They say that people who love each other stays together on rough times, helps dealing with anxiety issues. I could easily figure out that my boyfriend was distancing himself from me and I was wondering that we just had a very amazing trip together and could not understand the reason for his behavior. I decided to confront him, and it is then I came to know he was not sure about me. It broke me into million pieces and the isolation became difficult to bear. I remember a month full of anxiety, crying, sleeping late, trying to hold myself together. In India, most of the families are not very open regarding the intimate relationships, so talking to them about my problem was not even in picture. I did not even have enough space to cry, let me anxiety out. I called my friends almost every day until I got the strength to deal with this on my own. The only ways I knew of getting over a heartbreak was to go out, getting drunk with my friends, go for casual hookups. This time I had to confront a heartbreak rather than running away from it. I had to sit with my-self and listen over my emotions speaking loudly. After a month of waiting for his texts, calls, checking out his social media handles, checking over last seen, I decided to pull myself out of it dealing with the isolation altogether. I am an academically oriented person, so achieving small goals in a day makes me good about myself. For couple of days I tried to set very hard goals for myself. In the first week of lockdown month I registered myself for two courses on coursera and I finished them just in a week. I was working hard on myself and the sense of an outrageous performance consistently gave me the feeling of satisfaction. I stopped talking to my friends about it with the motivation to get over it all by myself. However, none of these helped with the anxieties I met almost every night. The days were normal and productive, but nights were equally harsh. No matter how much I forced myself to sleep it did not happen. Meanwhile the whole world was having rough time, but my heartbreak made it very difficult for me. People were taking 30 days challenges, working on their fitness or their hobbies, on the other hand I was barely able to do house chores. Pandemic situation however turned out to be blessing in disguise for me. After being 7 years in a relationship I completely lost myself, all my planning, my thoughts were derived from people I love. I desperately needed to work on my inner engineering rather than distracting myself by being more career orientated. I remember how I use to tell my friends to get over something until, I had to do the same, I realized the amount of strength it takes to just make first move. After days of crying, panicking, missing, and working hard to distract myself I decided to address these dark emotions rather than running from them. The very first thing I needed to be avoid late night hour thoughts, because 2 :00 am thoughts are the one which haunt you most and do not let you sleep peacefully. For this, I needed to change my entire schedule I was following from last couple of days. I read somewhere that most creative hours are either early morning hours or late-night hours. I have been a morning person before, so this was not very difficult for me. I started waking up at 6 AM in the morning and decided to do 30 minutes yoga and few minutes of meditation everyday followed by reading book for 1 hour every morning. I have always known the benefits of mediation and thought something to be easily adapted in daily life, but the very first day I was barely able to concentrate for 2 minutes. For first few days I would quit every time my thoughts started wandering while meditating. A friend of mine suggested me to use an alarm of at least 5 minutes and do not quit at the moment your thoughts wander rather try to bring your attention back in your inner circle. I started practicing the same and it worked, every time my thoughts would wander, I tried hard to bring them back and after couple of days I got a hold of it. Meditation and yoga helped me in a way I never imagined. It helped me to convert my frustration and anxiety into calmness and a positive energy. This time, I promised myself to maintain consistency because it is easy to start a new activity very enthusiastically but with time the intensity might decline. I did not start with very intensive yoga, rather I took an easy 30 days challenge and worked more on focusing my inner energy with the help of various asanas. I have always avoided working out in gym my entire life. My go to work out had been running or practicing kickboxing. For me, learning a skill set along with physically maintaining my body is very important therefore I have always chosen either sports or learning a martial art as a way of keeping my body in shape. Along with the physical benefits, I also believe the regular exercising have the tendency to fall into monotonous schedule but a physical training involving a skill set always plays a part of something we can look forward to everyday. However, yoga was unique from anything I did so far, it made me learn the meaning of self-awareness and balancing my focus. For every 30 minutes in morning I forgot everything that was messing up with my head, I was at a high place where

I was at peace. Day by day I started getting hold of every basic yoga posture and with time I understood the impact it has on the world and why thousands of people devote themselves to yoga lessons.

Though these activities helped me to calm down my mind but now it was time to deal with real issues inside me. We hardly sit with our self to realize what is going on inside us and evaluate our happiness as the measure of performance in life goals. The world stat shows that 60% of youngsters deals with mental issues those are mostly related to insecurities, loneliness, and fear of being alone. The modern world dating gives us many options but is not able to fill the gaps we are seeking out. In the generation of hookups, casual dating it is very easy to throw our insecurities in the form of casual sex or dating several people. However, it is very important to deal with the personal insecurities first to love yourself and all your flaws, it is only then one can welcome another human being into their life. The answer to the question: what your weakness" the kind we tell in interviews like time management, punctuality, it is more than that, for me it was developing the art of letting go. We have been at a place where we get hurt or hurting others. I had a good share of teenage relationships but there is one heartbreak which affects you to the core, if you are giver kind of person this will hurt. To my surprise I always thought I am a giver because I have too much love to give, I dive in into the relationship. But it is at the time of healing process I realized most of it came from me not being able to ever love myself enough to let go of the person. I sat almost every-day and asked myself certain questions why I was feeling like in a certain way other night. Earlier I had the tendency to distract myself with work or achieving career goals whenever I had to deal with an emotional situation like heartbreak. But a breakup should not be a motivation for that or moving on from someone is not. Every day, I found the need to achieve something to realize my worth. The day I do not achieve anything I started feeling frustrated and hating myself more. It is very important to give yourself the time to heal. That graph will not be ever linear, somedays I felt confident and other days same as day 1. Until you allow yourself to completely heal without distracting yourself with other works, you never would be able to let go of person and that will reflect in your future friendships or relationships but for that you will have to stop being scared about addressing your feeling though it might make you feel weak. However before becoming strong realizing your weak spots comes first. Pick up with small habits and do them falling in love with yourself takes twice a long time as for falling in love with another person. Moving on is just another form of intoxicating your heart and mind. You must feel sorry for yourself. By one month of my breakup I did all, I cried I shouted silently and all of that. But I allowed myself to be a mess before picking myself up and everyday told myself to get my shit together girl, I was my own therapist. Every day, I asked myself whether I want to feel the same way I felt every night before falling asleep. They say communication is the key, be communicative to yourself first and the one day you do not have to listen to anyone but your conscious.

No matter how bad the situation was for me, if was far better than the people experiencing in my country. India has around 60% of population involved in agriculture and small-scale business. This makes around 40% of people working as labors in the metropolitan cities. There were thousands of immigrants living away from their villages and families. As the lockdown was announced these people lost the source of income and had to suffer with basic necessities like paying their house rents and daily meals. In the developing nations, per hour wage in is not sufficient to fill empty stomachs for days. The chaos was across the country, when riches were celebrating pandemic as a break from their hectic life, poor were homeless and trying to feed their children and family. The government announced the fund of few crores for to help the people with below poverty line, but the help was reaching only to few people. It must not have been easy for government to help millions of people at the same time, but a part of system being corrupted also hindered the wellbeing of these people. There was not any preplan of evacuating labor workers stuck in other parts of the cities due to their work. Meanwhile government was evacuating NRIs stranded in other countries, but no transportation was arranged for the people with less privileges. This is when 1000 of labor workers decided to walk back their homes on foot for distances of around 1200 km. Few were travelling by cycles and few were travelling on foot holding their children and their belongings. I remember reading in a news that a girl covered the distance of 2000 km carrying her father on her bicycle and made it to her home in 20 days. Later she was called to one the biggest cycling competition firm for training. The world sure is opportunist, they find benefits in the struggles. Another news which shook me was of three men died on railway tracks who assumed that the trains were not running anymore and therefore decided to take a nap on railway tracks but they had no information that cargo trains were running. The lack of information and awareness killed three men. Sitting under my roof, with three meals in a day I realized the privileges I have. I had every source of entertainment at my home from internet to board games. I had my family with me, I was able to connect with my friends over video call and still I was cribbing about my boredom. Times like these make us empathize with the people who suffers and struggles to sustain. The hunger was not the only thing these people suffered; they suffered watching their kids die due to lack of water, their grandparents die with no resources of treatment. Consuming news everyday made me think to contribute to this cause in any form I can. There were a lot of donation options on the internet, many NGOs started online funding, even government opened an account dedicated to accepting huge donations from across the country. I had no job at that time, even though I had some savings, but I wanted to help directly. At same time, I came across an NGO named Indus action who was supporting the workers by connecting them to the departments helping with essential services like food, water, and income. This organization was very apt for me as I was to be supposed to make 50 calls from home and ask people if they were suffering with anything due to pandemic. Initially I was quite nervous with the fact that these people must be already feeling very hopeless with the government and listening to a someone with no direct solution might leave them feel frustrated with the whole system. We were given a 6 hours training to deal with people on call. The most important thing we were told to be empathize with the people and do not call like a call center person rather call them as their well wishers and friends. It was my first day of calling and I was supposed to use only Hindi, it is a common language in my state. Living outside of my home for around 6 years made me less confident in my regional language and it is when I realized while calling people that I need to work on my vocabulary. I got better day by day and started feeling very attached to the suffering families. I would not just do formality of asking few questions in order rather I tried to know them more and every-time asked them to call me at any hour if they face any issue. The volunteering work was not just limited to calls, sometimes if the person suffering from necessities is living close to the volunteer's residential area, he or she is supposed to decide to help them in person. I was confronted with the similar situation, where a group of people in a nearby village were not getting water supply for past one week. I had no knowledge of higher authorities who deal with water issues therefore I tried to research more and called every possible person in concern. The call was not sufficient, I somehow managed to visit the authority and explained them the importance of situation. After struggling for a while, they were ready to help and we left with a tank of water that village. On reaching there, my eyes were shocked looking at the miserable condition these people were living in. the only hope they had in their eyes was a bucket of water and as soon as the water tank stopped for supply, hundreds of people gathered to collect water breaking social distancing rule. It is impossible to follow rules when the hunger and thirst makes a person helpless. I am a person who loves to wander and idea of being stuck at a place is something I never thought of, but I was turning into a different person in the middle of this chaos. Every day I started feeling grateful for things I have, for the family I am spending time with, this was a blessing in disguise for me. Meanwhile when humans were merely able to survive, the animals outside were living their best lives ever. Initially the rumors were spread about animals being affected by virus and many households started abandoning their pets and there was nothing more than sad than those helpless lives. However very soon after the rumor WHO released statements confirming that the dogs and cats are not affected by virus. I remember the overwhelming feeling of watching videos of penguins roaming outside their zoo cage, few other animals in zoos could meet other type of animals. For the first time in years, humans were captured inside the houses and the animals were set free. I remember in month of May people had the sight of three tigers in a jungle near my village. The pain of being captured at one place made a lot of people empathize with animals who are captured and trained with cruelty. The number of people were joining animal protection organizations like PETA. Being a non-vegetarian, that month I came to terms of not eating animals anymore.

The three months were passed, and I was already picturing the life post pandemic, the new way of living, where self-care and conscious living comes first, where a rat race stops. A new world, where people are helping each other mentally, people are dropping off food on stranger's porches, restaurants are delivering free food to people, netizens are making sure that nobody is suffering with the mental issues and trying to make social groups to engage as many people, healthcare workers are putting their lives on stake to save thousands, families checking on neighbors and bachelors' living alone away from family, people singing for each in the balconies, eating together by sliding plates from one balcony to another , donations , gratitude, the world is getting better amidst the chaos. I have never seen the world at this best for the last few years. All I saw was people running for 9 – 5 jobs, weird frowns on the public commute, no contact policies with the neighbors. Although this is the worst pandemic since years, it is turning our world upside down. It is a new ray of hope in the direction of becoming better humans and save humanity. We have been doing so much harm to nature on the name of technology and industrial advancements, This is a reality check that if we want to survive on our planet we must abide by the rules of environment field technology inventions. Today we have the best transport, best cellphones, almost best of anything but still we are helpless.

With the months passing everyone started adapted the new life and more over started praising the new life. Few months back before pandemic, people would complain about almost everything from early morning traffics to their wives calling them everyday at work. I personally loved having my complete space and every time my family would call, I would end up hanging up within 15 to 20 minutes. Talking to them for hours, cracking jokes, talking about everyday life was something I thought they would never understand. Four months of living at home since past 6 years taught me everything from und=conditional love of my parents to the comfort of house I spent my childhood. The first month frustration turned out to be a beautiful bonding with my parents. I always claimed that living alone is the best thing in young days but so is staying with our parents. In India, usually children do not leave their parent's house until they find a job or a college in another city and this makes India a very family-oriented country. One might hate the fact of staying with parents supported by reasoning of being independent but at home you can create your own personal space. The idea of working from home was very annoying for me and every time I would switch place and find my space to focus. It took me around 3 weeks to settle down for a perfect spot where my entire focus was on my work and not on surrounding. I started by modifying my study table with some DIY ideas since I wanted to engage myself in a creative activity as well. I placed my favourite books on the table, print outs of my idols and a very small plant which I grew myself during the lockdown period. Just this little activity helped me shift my energy towards the things I wanted to do. With time I started taking two online space system courses and started reading a lot of blogs. One day, while sitting at the same table I tried to describe one of my experience through a blog. It was very first time I wrote something about myself. I never kept a journal neither I wrote letters for any of my loved ones therefore I was very conscious of someone reading it. I thought of sending to a friend without any intention of publicizing it. The very first remarks that came out of mouth were whether I wrote this blog out of emotions and I realized that is what writing is all about. Making other person feel your story, your emotions through the flow of words. I was very overwhelmed with my friend's response and I thought of getting it read from one or two more friends. To my surprise everyone connected with it. I did not care much about the literature rather I used a simple form of English while describing my emotions. After getting enough it proof-read, I gained some experience to upload my blog on a platform. I already had a membership of one of the blogging apps called medium, I made my profile and uploaded my first ever blog on it. I did not share it everywhere but only on the social media platforms where few people were able to read it. In the very day I received the positive response, but I was not sure whether I can write, or it barely came out as a candid writeup. However, I tried to write at least one blog every week for about three to four weeks and this was it. I started realizing the happiness I get penning down my thoughts. I started giving one hour every day to understand the skills and would implement them in my blogs. I have never known my side hustle, I never knew anything other than my course books, I had no special creative skill like dancing or singing but writing was my calling. I treated it as my 5- 9 job, I gave early hours to my writing and kept rest of the day for my academic work. I never considered myself a good writer because the only writing I knew was to use of very high-level vocabulary in the writeup. One consistent month of working and I got published with 2 top level publication on medium and one of my articles got curate by medium editors. This might not play a significance in top level writer's profile but for me as an amateur, it was enough to build a confidence in me. I never had the sense of achievement with my score card but getting positive results inside hustle started making me feel fulfilled.

To me spending this time at home turned out to be a time of realizing and reevaluating every decision I made in my life in last 20 years. Without this forced pause, I would be still running in the rat race of achievements. There was a time I also questioned my decision to go to Germany in the first place. No matter how much I fell in love with Berlin, but it has not felt like home since last year. My parents place gave me the feeling of belongingness I have been craving for and living with them made me realize that we have forgot the true meaning of unconditional love, the bonding we have with our closed ones. Almost every teenager today complains about parents' interference in their personal lives but what we do not realize is everything they do is out of love. My parents scolds me almost everyday for not waking up on time or being unorganized with my clothes, my mom makes me special dishes, my dad asks about my future plans, my brother annoys me but still loves me and late night bed talks with my sister are full of sharing secrets. I have been missing on these things since years and I am not ready to accept the fact that once again I have to move back because our world has hard wired us with following up the plans we set for us. In the pursuit of those goals we forget the pursuit of our happiness. Back in 60s the families use to live together, they shared their three-time meals, their sorrows and happiness together. Today we share our emotions on some drinks, sometimes with a stranger or a person whom we barely know. Socializing has changed its definition in today's world, its more about meeting people over meetups and dating apps rathe than establishing a real bond with people. If we don't approve of someone because of their looks or the way they dress or due to that fact they don't have anything in common with you, we tend to move on in the search of our new soulmate. The true bonds take time, patience, and nourishment, it could take years to establish a same bond with someone we have with our family.

Slowly and steadily lockdown period was coming to end in India and other parts of the world. Here in India we were entering into unlock phase 1 where government decided to remove few restrictions. It was 3rd day of unlock phase and I finally broke all the shackle and met my school friends again after 3 months. I made my special banana cake for them which I leaned during lockdown phase. I woke up very early that morning to spend maximum number of hours with them. We were not allowed to go to eat in restaurants therefore we planned a get together at one of my friend's place. We were joyous to see each other after a long time, we played cards, gossiped about old classmates, and talked about our ex-boyfriends. There were few walkways opened to residential path so we decided to go for a walk in the neighborhood, we could see some people walking with their kids after saw long. Everywhere we were watching people with smiling faces and less of tired faces. People were appreciating the freedom they were experiencing after so long. They were not just walking outside; they were enjoying every bit of fresh air. A few hours later I noticed the time, it was already 6 PM and for very first time in three months the day did not felt longer. As I came home, I laid down on my sofa thinking of the good times I had that day because in the end of day we all crave for little things that makes our day.

When the world started looking after each other, there were new situations coming to shake the world again and this time it was not a virus but a human form of virus. The pandemic is not ending any soon and world is already facing problems. In around 4th month of pandemic a news hit everyone's mind. A news in US of a black man getting murdered by a cop spread all over world fire. The racism towards black in America is not something new but this time it hit the rock bottom. A man held by the cop under his knee, was crying "I can't breathe, I can't breathe" and the cop along with other two cops didn't considered his life to be of any importance and few seconds later the man was choked to death. The entire scene happened in the middle of street, with hundreds of other vehicles passing, with a store write in front of street, with people walking on side paths, but no one cared to stop and get him rid of the man. The problem was not just with the cops but also with people who avoided the scenario and chosen to remain n shut. This time black people did not stay calm, they started raising their voices towards the cruelty they have been facing since years. Thousands of people came down on streets for protests starting from US to Europe and later all over the world. It became a big resistance movement from the month of June. everyone seems to have forgotten about the social distancing rules, the infection of virus, the world got angry and wanted justice for a man who was brutally killed. It might not be the correct decision at that time, but when police were supposed to help people without any racism they did exactly opposite, when world should have been more humble and supportive towards people the people were getting murdered. The moment like these do not wait for a pandemic to end, it rather shows what a brutally unemphatic world we live in. There are thousands out there, who found the pandemic as an opportunity to earn profits, to play politically, to spread hatred. India started facing border issues with China and in addition 4 army officers got killed in Kashmir by terrorist. When all the countries needed each other's helping hand, economic politics were being played. China being the largest manufacturer sent testing kits two 4 nations and those nations were not able to do testing as required. On the other hand, America cut down its funding to WHO asserted by the reason of WHO supported China in its dirty secret of hiding first few cases due to deadly virus. India has largest democracy in the world and a country with the greatest number of religious conflicts. Even pandemic did not stop this conflict and a group of Muslims was being targeted for spreading pandemic in India. These were the people who sheltered themselves in a large mosque past a huge religious gathering including some foreigners and higher authorities of mosque did not informed any health authority unless everyone was evacuated from there to their homelands. When the focus shall have been more on identifying the culprits, the entire focus was shifted on targeting Muslim community and spread hatred towards them via news channels and social medias. This explains that real world is not full of humanity, everyone is divided, we are robots being operated by the people in power. Same goes for various organizations. A friend of mine told me about her situation of how her company did not pay her anything for work from home and deducted the amount from her paid leaves. I remember in the first month of pandemic my mother discussing with my father that they shouldn't pay anything for the house help since she is on holiday however no one can call a forced holiday due to pandemic a holiday. I explained my mother that you would have reacted in a different manner if our organization were not paying us for working from home or our government would not be helping us out with the economic situations. Somehow, she got convinced to pay her 60% of her usual pay. On the other hand, few families in our locality decided to send food thrice a week for our and labor workers loving nearby.

At around the same time India was hit by cyclone, killing hundreds of people in eastern part of India followed by a loss of around lakhs; this was another situation where people needed to get their lives back more than worrying about pandemic, huge amount of donations were paid to build the city and start again before infections hit them hard. The month of May and June came up with storm of killing people due to three disasters at the same time and the days were not getting any better. After three months of battling with pandemic now world seems ready to fight against pandemic.

The European countries eased the lockdown restrictions. People started coming out on streets and only of them were following social distancing. The world was not safe, but people seem to care more about their leisure than the infection. Meanwhile the countries were still trying to develop vaccines but now the world started getting normal due to economic loss. Slowly restaurants were opening, people were visiting lakes, enjoying the summers but who knows when the second wave is going to hit the world again.

Looking at the world getting normal I also started planning my trip back to Berlin, though international travel was not started but there were few evacuation flights been run by Indian government. I wanted to go back and earn money to have a hold on my finances so did not hesitated to book this ticket was a bit more than the normal fare. The day I booked my ticket, I felt a sense of anxiety running in me. That day I could not sleep whole night. The past three months, staying close to family was very nurturing for me and this time I had to step again into the real world and face it again. The going back felt like leaving a homely and comforting feeling behind, though I started considering Berlin as my home but this time I was scared to feel the loneness Berlin offers to youngsters. There are many activities to join, many clubs to be member of, hangout buddies for a day but the city still feel lonely. No matter how much I prepared myself to face my demons alone, it felt back to the day 1, the anxiety was really bumping me hard. During the last few days, my Ex started calling me and told me his urge to spend some time with me before leaving. I agreed on the idea thinking that I am moved on and meeting one last time would not be a big deal. However more I analyzed, the more I realized that he wanted some last action and my conscious did not allowed me to be a part of his need. It is then I realized I was still not moved on but just detached from this person, however I choose to stay back and continue working on myself. When I was fighting my own battles a death of very renounced person in our Bollywood due to suicide shook the entire country. He was the man who would inspire thousands of children though his space talks, he had 50 things to do in his bucket list and was one of the best actors we got in Bollywood. His death was a direct reflection of humanity and a lesson that we have come so fat that we have forgotten the importance of little things in life. The mental illness was drastically increasing during pandemic, and this was not getting any better with days passing. This news made me to checkup my friends and just listen to them about their problems. That day, I remember releasing the times when I did not paid attention to a friend who was sad and shrugged the conversation thinking that the person is just over thinking. The fear of losing them put me in the position to reach out to my closed ones every now and then. Sometimes our close friends put on a smiling face and hide their demons inside which we are not able to be recognizing and the pandemic was making it worse. Same day on his death I asked my mom that why do you think the mental illness existed very less in your time but its escalating in today's time among youngsters. One answer she gave really hit me hard was that in her time there was not any expectations from the 10 year of 5 year later plan. They lived in the environment which was surrounded by loved ones and every day they were nourished with care and compassion. Today we all are lost in the pursuit of our goals and when we reach the top, we crave to find ourselves or someone who would hold us in bad and good times.

Today, I am going to Berlin in another 2 weeks but this time it feels very different to leave home. I have not felt that ache in my heart before leaving my childhood house since felt years. I am reliving each corner of the house, where I healed myself, where I promised myself a transformation, the beautiful lawn where I spent evenings reading my favourite books. In last 4 months I did not just passed time, I lived the time. I lived the time doing things that I love since I was young. I lived my life when I created a sketch of a princes, when I colored the galaxy and listened to the favourite songs for hours. After so many years if felt good to be home but leaving was equally hard. I planned an activity for every day I these two weeks including cycling to my favourite spots, meeting my school friends. My yoga practice is still on and for the very first time I have been consistent for so long, I feel less frustrated and more compassionate towards my family members. In these two weeks I promised I am just not going back to normal life, going to work and stay busy all day rather I am taking a new way of living with myself. In the past few months, I learned the art of letting go, I gave priority to my mental health. The old me would think about the financial burden., the work stress and would not be compassionate but new me is leaving all the toxicity behind. Personally, this pandemic was a turning point for me and for so many other people. People have started understanding the importance of spreading positivity in the world, people are holding up each other, the world is healing in ways we never though of. I wonder if two years from today we are living a new normal where there is more of humanity. The world does not need more successful people and new products for comfort, the world needs more peacemakers in the form of human beings who does not kill their own and other species on planet. The world needs its equilibrium, it needs clean air and millions of trees instead of million of 50 story buildings. Every generation comes with a change, new civilization will be formed but it should not be on account of destruction of our own Planet. We must move forward but our priories shall remain intact, our principles and values should not come after our urge of money or success. I hope for a new normal once this pandemic is over, a world with new start.

IMPRINT

All rights reserved

Mindful Publishing

by

TTENTION Inc.

Trolley SQ 20c
Wilmington
DE 19806

www.ingramcontent.com/pod-product-compliance
Lightning Source LLC
Chambersburg PA
CBHW050323220526
45465CB00005B/2113